CW00691034

Lean and (

Life

50 Healthy Recipes to

Rebuild Your Body and

Get a Healthier Life

By

Spoons of Happiness

Table of Contents

Introduction 8

Chapter 1: Snacks Recipes 11

    1. White Chocolate Snack Mix 12

    2. Extra Easy Hummus 13

    3. No-Bake Energy Bites 14

    4. Baked Oatmeal Breakfast Bars 15

    5. Microwave Popcorn 17

Chapter 2: Breakfast Recipes....................... 18

    6. Pumpkin Spice Protein Drink........................... 19

    7. Chai-Spiced Oatmeal with Mango 20

    8. Skinny Pepper, Tomato & Ham Omelet 21

    9. Refried Beans without the Refry.......................23

    10. Banana Yogurt Pots.......................................25

Chapter 3: Lunch Recipes.............................26

    11. Kappa (Tapioca)..27

    12. Green Pea Upma (Indian recipe) 29

    13. Spicy Papadum (Indian Recipe)......................31

14. River Sole for Your Soul 32

15. Hassel Back Sweet Potatoes 34

16. Mustard-Parmesan Whole Roasted Cauliflower

....36

Chapter 4: Dinner Recipes 39

17. Double Crunch Honey Garlic Pork Chops........ 40

18. Cauliflower Chowder...42

19. Zucchini Lasagna..45

20. Lemon Garlic Dump Chicken 48

21. Mushroom-Stuffed Cabbage Rolls 50

22. Insanely Easy Vegetarian Chili 53

Chapter 5: Soups Recipes 55

23. Absolutely Ultimate Potato Soup.....................56

24. Fresh Asparagus Soup 58

25. Healing Cabbage Soup 60

26. Avgolemono 62

27. Chunky Chicken Noodle Soup 63

28. Spaetzle and Chicken Soup.............................. 64

Chapter 6: Vegan Recipes 67

29. Easy Tofu Shirataki Stir-Fry Style 68

30. Vegan Stuffed Peppers with Rice...................... 69

31. Pressure Cooker Sambar (Indian Lentil Curry) 72

32. Homemade Vegetable Sushi 75

33. Easy Creamy Vegan Mushroom Risotto...........76

34. Easy, Healthy Falafel 79

Chapter 7: Meat Dishes................................81

35. Meat in its Juices... 82

36. Classic and Simple Meat Lasagna................... 84

37. Restaurant-Style Taco Meat Seasoning 86

38. Meat-Lover's Slow Cooker Spaghetti Sauce 90

39. Good New Orleans Creole Gumbo...................92

40. Chef John's Italian Meatballs 96

Chapter 8: Salad Recipes 99

41. Warm Green Bean and Potato Salad with Goat
Cheese 100

42. Warm Bok Choy, Beet and Feta Salad............102

43. Arugula Salad with Bacon and Butternut Squash
....104

44. Roasted Lettuce, Radicchio, and Endive 105

45. Warm Thai Kale Salad 108

46. Maple Cannellini Bean Salad with Baby Broccoli and Butternut Squash 110

Chapter 9: Dessert Recipes 113

47. Frozen Blueberry Yogurt Pops 114

48. Cinnamon Gelatin Salad 115

49. Almond Ice 116

50. Cranberry Apple Gelatin Mold 117

Conclusion 119

Introduction

Losing weight is a gradual process that combines at least three factors: diet, exercise, or moderate physical activity and control of emotional factors such as stress and anxiety. In this sense, the Lean and Green diet is oriented towards the gradual adoption of healthy eating habits combined with moderate exercise and the advice of a coach and support groups. Additionally, this diet promotes the consumption of low-calorie foods and low-carbohydrate home-cooked meals that will contribute to weight loss.

In principle, the diet consists of a combination of pre-packaged products called "Fuelings", which have controlled carbohydrates and calories along with lean proteins and non-starchy vegetables. In this way, an intake of 80 to 100 grams of carbohydrates per day is obtained together with a low caloric intake of 800 to 1000 calories.

Gradually replacing the "Fuelings" with a "Lean & Green" meal consisting of meat, vegetables, and balanced fat will allow you to feel satisfied and without cravings. Once the plan is completed, it is expected that by substituting packaged meals with other lean and green food, you will adopt better eating habits for life, coupled with moderate physical exercise and the support of your coach.

The idea is to eat six or more mini-meals a day between "fuelings" and home-cooked meals. These meals include bars, shakes, cookies, cereals, soup, and mashed potatoes, all of which have soy protein or whey protein as the first ingredient.

The above foods are combined with 3 servings of non-starchy vegetables, 5-7 ounces of lean protein such as tuna, chicken, egg whites, turkey or soy, and no more than 2 servings of balanced fat.

The Green and Lean diet works on the principle of decreased carbohydrate intake, in which, the body begins to use alternate fuel sources such as protein and healthy fats and begins to burn fat. Nutritionists always state that it is better to eat several times a day in moderate amounts than to eat three times and then binge eat as this maintains satiety longer and the body burns more this way.

The eating plan is aimed at consuming 800-1000 calories a day in six controlled meal portions. Another of its benefits is the control of blood pressure by decreasing salt intake. Also, the Green and Lean diet can be maintained over time by avoiding hunger and cravings that make us give up on dieting.

This book will guide you on the road to weight loss and better health to achieve the ideal weight you have longed for, but don't forget that it requires a high degree of commitment.

Chapter 1: Snacks Recipes

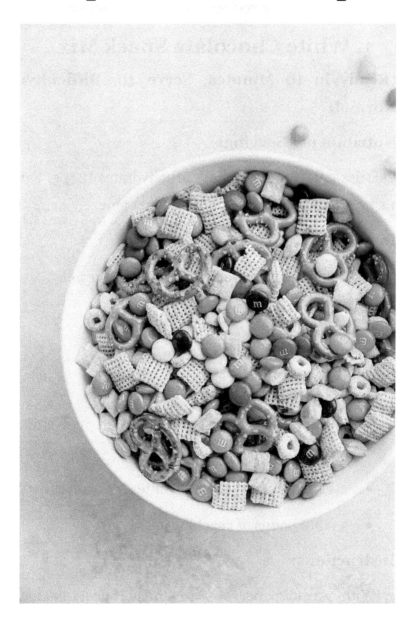

In this chapter, we are going to give you some delicious and mouthwatering recipes on Octavia Snacks recipes.

1. White Chocolate Snack Mix

(Ready in 10 Minutes, Serve 40, Difficulty: Normal)

Nutrition per Serving:

Calories 240, Protein 4.5 g, Carbohydrates 18.3 g, Fat 12.7 g, Cholesterol 4.7mg, Sodium 262.3mg.

Ingredients:

- 1(10 ounces) package of mini twist pretzels
- 5 cups of toasted oat cereal
- 5 cups of crispy corn cereal squares
- 2 cups of salted peanuts
- 1(14 ounces) package of candy-coated milk chocolate pieces
- 2(11 ounces) packages of white chocolate chips
- 3 tablespoons of vegetable oil

Instructions:

1. With waxed paper or parchment, line 3 baking sheets. Set aside.

2. Combine mini pretzels, toasted oat cereal, crispy squares of corn cereal, salted peanuts, and candy-coated chocolate bits in a large bowl. Set aside.

3. Heat chips and oil in a microwave-safe bowl over medium-high heat for 2 minutes, stirring once.

5. Microwave for 10 seconds on high, stirring until smooth. Pour over the mixture of cereal and combine properly.

6. Spread over ready-made baking sheets. Cool, and break apart.

7. Store in an airtight jar.

2. Extra Easy Hummus

(Ready in 10 Minutes, Serve 2, Difficulty: Easy)

Nutrition per Serving:

Calories 118, Protein 3.7 g, Carbohydrates 16.5 g, Fat 4.4 g, Cholesterol 0mg, Sodium 501.9mg.

Ingredients:

- 1(15 ounces) can of garbanzo beans, drained and liquid reserved

- 1 clove of garlic, crushed

- 2 teaspoons of ground cumin

- ½ teaspoon of salt

- 1 tablespoon of olive oil

Instructions:

1. Mix the garbanzo beans, salt, garlic, and olive oil in a blender or food processor. Blend at a low level, adding the reserved bean liquid gradually.

2. Until they obtain the required consistency.

3. No-Bake Energy Bites

(Ready in 30 Minutes, Serve 2, Difficulty: Normal)

Nutrition per Serving:

Calories 219, Protein 2.5 g, Carbohydrates 10.6 g, Fat 5.3 g, Cholesterol 0mg, Sodium 27.9mg.

Ingredients:

- 1 cup of rolled oats

- ½ cup of mini semi-sweet chocolate chips

- ½ cup of ground flax seed

- ½ cup of crunchy peanut butter

- ⅓ cup of honey

- 1 teaspoon of vanilla extract

Instructions:

1. In a bowl, mix oats, flax seeds, chocolate chips, peanut butter, sugar, and vanilla extract, and use your hands to shape balls.

2. On a baking sheet, place energy bites and freeze once set, nearly for 1 hour.

4. Baked Oatmeal Breakfast Bars

(Ready in 1 Hour and 5 Minutes, Serve 8, Difficulty: Normal)

Nutrition per Serving:

Calories 118, Protein 5.3 g, Carbohydrates 16.2 g, Fat 6.7 g, Cholesterol 48.9mg, Sodium 270.6mg.

Ingredients:

- 2 cups of old-fashioned rolled oats
- ⅓ cup of packed brown sugar
- 1 tablespoon of white sugar
- 1 ½ teaspoon of baking powder
- ½ teaspoon of salt

- ½ teaspoon of ground cinnamon

- 1 cup of milk

- 2 eggs

- 2 tablespoons of canola oil

- 1 teaspoon of vanilla extract

Instructions:

1. Preheat the oven to 350 degrees Fahrenheit (176 degrees Celsius). Grease an 8-inch square pan.

2. In a bowl, add the oatmeal, baking powder, brown sugar, white sugar, salt, and cinnamon. In a separate bowl, whisk together the milk, canola oil, eggs, and vanilla extract.

3. Stir the egg mixture into the oat mixture until well mixed, set aside for around 20 minutes until the flavors blend. Spread the blended oats into the prepared square pan.

4. Bake in the preheated oven for around 30 minutes, until the sides are golden brown.

5. Microwave Popcorn

(Ready in 5 Minutes, Serve 4, Difficulty: Normal)

Nutrition per Serving:

Calories 137, Protein 4.1 g, Carbohydrates 14.6 g, Fat 3.1 g, Cholesterol 0mg, Sodium 388.6mg.

Ingredients:

- ½ cup of unpopped popcorn

- 1 teaspoon of vegetable oil

- ½ teaspoon of salt, or to taste

Instructions:

1. Mix the unpopped popcorn and oil in a cup or small bowl. Pour the coated corn into a lunch bag of brown paper and sprinkle it with salt. To seal in the ingredients, fold the top of the bag over twice.

2. Cook for 2 ½-3 minutes in the microwave at full power, or before you hear a delay of around 2 seconds between pops.

3. Open the bag cautiously to prevent steam, then pour it into a serving bowl.

Chapter 2: Breakfast Recipes

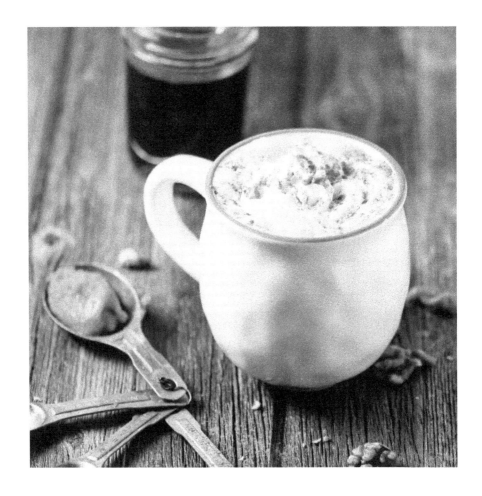

In this chapter, we are going to give you some delicious and mouthwatering recipes on Octavia Breakfast recipes.

6. Pumpkin Spice Protein Drink

(Ready in 10 Minutes, Serve 6, Difficulty: Easy)

Nutrition per Serving:

Calories 280, Protein 22 g, Carbohydrates 45.6 g, Fat 3 g, Cholesterol 6.3mg, Sodium 191.8mg.

Ingredients:

- 2 bananas, sliced and frozen
- ½ cup of canned pumpkin
- 2 dates, pitted
- 1 scoop of vanilla protein powder
- ½ teaspoon of vanilla extract
- 1 pinch of ground nutmeg
- 1 pinch of ground cinnamon
- 1 pinch of ground cloves
- 1 pinch of ground ginger

Instructions:

Blend almond milk, pumpkin, bananas, dates, protein powder, cinnamon, cloves, vanilla extract, and nutmeg in a blender, and ginger together until smooth.

7. Chai-Spiced Oatmeal with Mango

(Ready in 13 Minutes, Serve 2-3, Difficulty: Easy)

Nutrition per Serving:

Calories 236, Protein 6 g, Carbohydrates 10 g, Fat 4 g, Fiber 5.5 g.

Ingredients:

- 3 cups water
- 1 cup steel-cut oats
- ½ teaspoon vanilla
- Dash of cinnamon
- Dash of ginger
- Dash of cloves
- Dash of cardamom
- Dash of salt
- ½ mango, cut into pieces

Instructions:

1. In the pressure cooker, mix the water with the oats.

2. Get the cover closed.

3. Click 'manual,' then cook on high pressure for 3 minutes.

4. Hit "cancel" as the beeper rings, then wait for the energy to come down naturally.

5. Place the lid open and stir well.

6. Season and taste.

7. Divide and add sliced mango into even servings.

8. Skinny Pepper, Tomato & Ham Omelet

(Ready in 15 Minutes, Serve 6, Difficulty: Normal)

Nutrition per Serving:

Calories 206, Protein 21 g, Carbohydrates 5 g, Fat 12 g, Saturates 3 g, Sugars 5 g, Fiber 1 g, Salt 1.21 g.

Ingredients:

- 2 whole eggs

- 3 egg whites

- 1 teaspoon of olive oil

- 1 red pepper, deseeded and finely chopped

- 2 spring onions, white and green parts kept separate and finely chopped

- Few slices of wafer-thin extra-lean ham, shredded

- 25 g of reduced-fat mature cheddar cheese

To Serve (optional):

- Wholemeal toast

- 1-2 chopped fresh tomatoes

Ingredients:

1. Mix some seasoning with the eggs and egg whites and put aside.

2. Heat the oil and cook the pepper for 3-4 minutes in a medium non-stick frying pan.

3. Throw the spring onions in the white parts and cook for a further 1 minute.

4. Pour in the eggs and cook until almost completely set, over medium heat.

5. Sprinkle on the ham and cheese and continue to cook until just put in the middle, or if you like it more done, flash it under a hot grill.

6. Serve with the green portion of the spring onion scattered on top, the sliced tomato, and some wholemeal toast straight from the pan.

9. Refried Beans without the Refry

(Ready in 8 Hours and 15 Minutes, Serve 15, and Difficulty: Normal)

Nutrition per Serving:

Calories139, Protein 8.5 g, Carbohydrates 25.4 g, Fat 0.5 g, Cholesterol 0mg, Sodium 784.7mg.

Ingredients:

- 1 onion, peeled and halved
- 3 cups of dry pinto beans, rinsed
- ½ fresh jalapeno pepper, seeded and chopped
- 2 tablespoons of minced garlic
- 5 teaspoons of salt
- 1 ¾ teaspoon of fresh ground black pepper

- ⅛ teaspoon of ground optional

- 9 cups of water

Instructions:

1. In a slow cooker, put the onion, rinsed beans, jalapeno, garlic, salt, pepper, and cumin together. To mix, pour in the water and stir. Cook for 8 hours on high flame, add more water as needed.

2. Strain the beans and conserve the oil. To achieve the desired consistency, mash the beans with a potato masher, by adding the water as needed.

10. Banana Yogurt Pots

(Ready in 30 Minutes, Serve 6, Difficulty: Easy)

Nutrition per Serving:

Calories 230, Protein 7 g, Carbohydrates 40 g, Fat 6 g, Saturates 1 g, Sugars 39 g, Fiber 1 g, Salt 0.23 g.

Ingredients:

- 1 (x-side) tub of thick yogurt

- 3-4 bananas, cut into chunks

- 4 tablespoons of sort dark brown sugar

- 25 g of toasted and chopped walnuts

Instructions:

1. Dollop approximately 1 tablespoon of yogurt into 4 little glasses at the bottom.

2. Add the banana layer and some more yogurt. Until the glasses are full, repeat the layers.

3. Scatter over the sugar and nuts and leave for 20 minutes in the refrigerator before the sugar has dissolved.

Chapter 3: Lunch Recipes

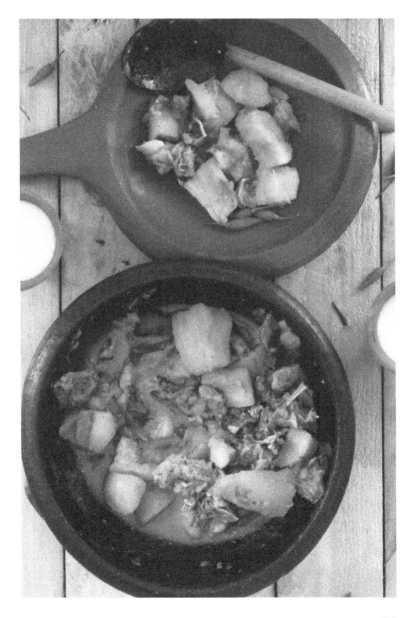

In this chapter, we are going to give you some delicious and mouthwatering recipes on Octavia Lunch recipes.

11. Kappa (Tapioca)

(Ready in 40 Minutes, Serve 6, Difficulty: Normal)

Nutrition per Serving:

Calories 100, Protein 0 g, Carbohydrates 26 g, Fat 0 g, Fiber 0 g, Sugar 0 g.

Ingredients:

- 2 Tapioca, cubed

- Tapioca water to cook

- Salt, to taste

To Grind:

- 1 Coconut

- 1 cumin seed

- 2 clove of garlic

- 1-2 green chili

- ¼-1/2 teaspoon of turmeric powder

- Salt, to taste

- Enough water to grind into a coarse paste

For Tempering:

- 2 tablespoons of coconut oil/vegetable oil

- 1 teaspoon of mustard seeds

- 3 small onions, finely chopped

- 3 red dry whole chili

- 1 sprig of curry leaves

Instructions:

1. Peel off the tapioca, cut it into cubes, and wash it under running water.

2. Boil the tapiocas until tender and well cooked, along with water and a little salt.

3. Drain and keep the water aside.

4. Grind ingredients in a blender to a coarse paste.

5. Add the cooked tapiocas as well as the ground paste into a large saucepan.

6. Cook until the gravy begins to thicken and is well mixed for around 5-10 minutes. You could use a wooden spoon to mash the tapiocas gently if you want.

7. Remove from the heat and cover aside.

8. Over medium heat, heat a small pan and add oil.

9. Add the mustard seeds as the oil gets hot and let it splutter.

10. Add the small sliced onions and cook them for a few minutes.

11. Add the dried red chilies and the curry leaves and cook before the onions turn brown.

12. Pour this mixture on the cooked tapioca.

13. For some time, leave the tapioca covered so that the tempering flavors will get into the bowl.

14. Along with your favorite fish curry, serve warm.

12. Green Pea Upma (Indian recipe)

(Ready in 25 Minutes, Serve 4, Difficulty: Easy)

Nutrition per Serving:

Calories 224, Protein 7 g, Carbohydrates 36 g, Fat 5 g.

Ingredients:

- 1 cup of roasted semolina

- ¼ cup of green peas

- 1 onion, finely chopped

- 2 green chilies, finely chopped
- 2 cups of hot water

For Tempering:

- 1 tablespoon of extra virgin olive oil
- ¾ teaspoon of mustard seeds
- 1 sprig of curry leaves
- 1 sprig ginger, grated
- Salt, to taste

For Garnishing:

- 2 sprigs of fresh coriander leaves (Optional)
- ½ tablespoon of boiled peas
- 1 sprig of curry leaves (cooked)

Instructions:

1. In a thick bottomed pan, heat oil and add mustard seeds. Let them crackle.

2. Add the curry leaves and grated ginger, and cook before the ginger's raw aroma disappears.

3. Now add the finely chopped onion, cook until smooth, add the green chilies, and cook for 2 minutes.

4. Now add the gently roasted semolina, add the green peas, cook, and add the hot water for 2 minutes.

5. To taste, add the salt. Stir to avoid lumps forming.

6. Cover it now and cook on a very slow heat until all the water is absorbed and the green peas and semolina are cooked.

7. Serve hot with sliced leaves of coriander or grated fresh coconut.

13. Spicy Papadum (Indian Recipe)

(Ready in 25 Minutes, Serve 6, Difficulty: Easy)

Nutrition per Serving:

Calories: 76, Protein 1.6 g, Carbohydrates 7 g, Fiber 2.8 g, Fat 0.3 g.

Ingredients:

- 1 cup tomato, chopped

- 1 cup onion, chopped

- 1 tablespoon of chopped coriander leaves

- 2 tbsp Lemon

- 1 teaspoon of salt

- 1 teaspoon of pepper

- Papadum

Instructions:

1. In a mug, mix the vegetables with the lemon juice, salt, and pepper. Take the papadums and cook them deep in a wok until they are crispy and crunchy. Put fried Papadum in a dish and uniformly place the spices and veggie mixture over it.

2. Serve with your favorite cold beer.

14. River Sole for Your Soul

(Ready in 50 Minutes, Serve 6, Difficulty: Normal)

Nutrition per Serving:

Calories 186, Protein 17.1 g, Carbohydrate 0 g, Fat 1.9 g, Sodium 95mg, Potassium 230mg.

Ingredients:

- 1 kg of sole fillet

- 5-10 large shrimps (Optional)

- 1 kg of peeled, sliced potatoes

- 3 onions, sliced

- 5 cloves of garlic, chopped

- ½ red/ green capsicum

- Parsley or coriander

- Few dashes of hot sauce

- 1 teaspoon of paprika

- 1 cup of olive oil

- 50 ml of white wine

- Rock salt, to taste

- Toasted garlic bread

Instructions:

1. Place the sliced onions, garlic, tomatoes, coriander, peppers, or parsley, sliced potatoes, and fish in a saucepan, forming layers.

2. In the upper layer, put the sliced onions and peppers, paprika, and salt. Evenly spread the olive oil over the layers.

3. Add seasoning and white wine, and a little water until all layers are set.

4. Cover the pan to get it to a boil.

5. Do not ever stir this dish,

6. Cover the pan and let it cook on a low flame. Once the potato is cooked, check that it is ready for serving.

7. Serve this stew with toasted garlic bread, so the soup appears rich and soupy.

15. Hassel Back Sweet Potatoes

(Ready in 1 Hour. and 10 Minutes, Serve 4, Difficulty: Normal)

Nutrition per Serving:

Calories 226, Protein 3 g, Carbs 40 g, Fat 6 g.

Ingredients:

- 4 medium sweet potatoes
- 6 tablespoons of butter, unsalted

- 1/3 cup of brown sugar

- 1 teaspoon of pure vanilla extract

- ½ teaspoons of ground cinnamon

- ½ teaspoons of Himalayan pink salt/rock salt

Instructions:

1. In the oven center, place an oven rack and preheat the oven to 218 degree Celsius (425 degrees Fahrenheit).

2. To give it a flat surface to stand on as you slice it, shave a thin sliver from one side of each potato. Make thin slices about 1/16-inch thick into the potato, stopping before cutting all the way through.

3. On a separate sheet of foil, place each potato. To seal them, shape the foil around the potatoes but leave the tops open and exposed.

4. On a rimmed baking sheet, place the potatoes.

5. Melt the butter over medium-high heat in a small skillet, stirring periodically, until browned and nutty, for 2- 3 minutes.

6. Stir in the brown sugar, vanilla, salt, and cinnamon. Over the potatoes, drizzle the butter mixture and pinch the foil together on top to seal the potato inside.

7. Bake for 45 minutes, then leave for a few moments to cool down. Remove the potatoes from the foil, place them on a serving dish, and drizzle each foil packet with the leftover sauce.

8. Sprinkle with some nuts as you serve.

16. Mustard-Parmesan Whole Roasted Cauliflower

(Ready in 1 Hour and 5 Minutes, Serve 2, Difficulty: Normal)

Nutrition per Serving:

Calories 107, Protein 2.5 g, Carbohydrates 6.2 g, Fat 8.9 g, Sodium 745mg, Potassium 189mg.

Ingredients:

- 2 large cauliflowers
- 1 clove of garlic, halved
- ¼ cup of olive oil

- 4 tablespoons of Dijon mustard

- Kosher salt

- Freshly ground of black pepper

- ½ cup of fresh parsley leaves, chopped

- ¼ cup of parmesan, grated

- Lemon wedges

Instructions:

1. In the bottom of the oven, place an oven rack and preheat to 232 Celsius (450 degrees Fahrenheit). Line a sheet with foil for baking.

2. Remove the leaves from the cauliflower, then trim the stem flush with the head's bottom, so the cauliflower sits flat on the prepared baking sheet.

3. With the sliced garlic, rub the outside of each head.

4. In a small bowl, whisk together the oil, 3 tablespoons of mustard, ½ teaspoon of salt, and a few tiny pieces of black pepper.

5. On the prepared baking sheet, place the cauliflower and brush the whole outside and inside with the mustard-oil mixture.

6. Roast the cauliflower until it is nicely charred and tender, 50 minutes to 1 hour (a long skewer inserted in the center of the cauliflower can pass through easily). Let them rest for a couple of minutes.

7. Meanwhile, in a small bowl, combine the parsley and the parmesan. Brush with the remaining one tablespoon mustard the outside of the roasted cauliflower heads all over and generously sprinkle the Parmesan mixture.

Chapter 4: Dinner Recipes

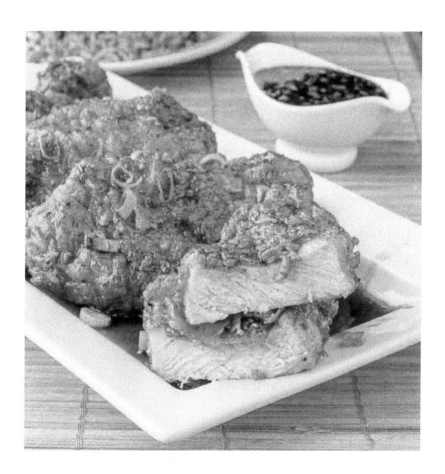

In this chapter, we are going to give you some delicious and mouthwatering recipes on Octavia Dinner recipes.

17. Double Crunch Honey Garlic Pork Chops

(Ready in 30 Minutes, Serve 4, Difficulty: Normal)

Nutrition per Serving:

Calories 336, Protein 33 g, Carbohydrates 55 g, Total Fat 22 g, Cholesterol 131mg, Sodium 251mg, Fiber 2 g, Sugar 47 g.

Ingredients:

- 6 center loin pork chops, well-trimmed

- 1 cup of flour

- 2 teaspoon of salt

- 1 1/2 tablespoon of ground ginger

- 2 teaspoons of black pepper

- 1 tablespoon of ground nutmeg

- 1 teaspoon of ground thyme

- 1/2 teaspoon of cayenne pepper

- 1 teaspoon of ground sage

- 1 tablespoon of paprika

- 2 eggs

- 4 tablespoons of water

For the Honey Garlic Sauce:

- 2 tablespoons of olive oil

- 3–4 cloves of garlic, minced

- 1 cup of honey

- ¼ cup of soy sauce (Low-sodium version is best)

- 1 teaspoon of ground black pepper

Instructions:

1. Sift the rice, salt, black pepper, ground ginger, thyme, nutmeg, sage paprika, and cayenne pepper together.

2. By whisking the eggs and water together, make an egg wash.

3. Season salt and pepper with the pork chops, then dip the meat into the flour and spice mixture. Dip the chop into the egg wash and then into the flour and spice mix for the final time, squeezing the mix into the meat to make good contact.

4. On the stove, heat a skillet with around half an inch of canola oil covering the bottom. Here, you want to carefully monitor the temperature so that the chops do not brown too fast.

5. Before dipping the cooked pork chops into the honey garlic sauce, drain for a few minutes on a wire rack. With noodles or rice, serve.

To make the Honey Garlic Sauce:

1. Add 2 tablespoons of olive oil and sliced garlic to a medium saucepan. To soften the garlic, cook over medium heat, but do not let it brown.

2. Add the honey, black pepper, and soy sauce.

3. For 5-10 minutes, boil together, remove from the heat and allow to cool for a few minutes. Watch this cautiously as it simmers because it can very easily foam up over the pot.

18. Cauliflower Chowder

(Ready in 45 Minutes, Serve 6, Difficulty: Normal)

Nutrition per Serving:

Calories 129, Protein 5.4 g, Carbohydrates 16 g, Fat 5.5 g, Sodium 408mg, Potassium 418mg, Sugars 4.1 g.

Ingredients:

- 4 slices of bacon, diced
- 2 tablespoons of unsalted butter
- 2 cloves of garlic, minced
- 1 onion, diced
- 2 carrots, peeled and diced
- 2 stalks of celery, diced
- 1/4 cup of all-purpose flour
- 4 cups of chicken broth
- 1 cup of 2% milk
- 1 head of cauliflower, roughly chopped
- 1 bay leaf
- Kosher salt and freshly ground black pepper, to taste
- 2 tablespoons of chopped fresh parsley leaves

Instructions:

1. Over medium heat, heat a big stockpot or Dutch oven. Add bacon and cook for around 6-8 minutes, until brown and crispy. Transfer to a paper towel-lined tray set aside.

2. In the stockpot, melt the butter. Add the onion, garlic, carrots, and celery. Cook for around 3-4 minutes, stirring periodically, until tender. Stir in the bay leaf and cauliflower. Cook for about 3-4 minutes, stirring periodically, until barely crisp-tender.

3. Whisk in the flour for around 1 minute, until lightly browned. Gradually whisk in the chicken broth and milk and cook for around 3-4 minutes, whisking continuously, until slightly thickened.

4. Bring to a boil, reduce heat and simmer until tender, around 12-15 minutes, and season to taste with salt and pepper. If the chowder is too thick, add more milk until the desired consistency is achieved, if necessary.

5. Serve immediately, garnished, if desired, with bacon and parsley.

19. Zucchini Lasagna

(Ready in 2 Hours, Serve 8, Difficulty: Hard)

Nutrition per Serving:

Calories: 275, Protein 26 g Carbohydrates 13 g, Fat 13 g, Saturated Fat 7 g, Cholesterol 84mg, Sodium 648mg, Fiber 2.5 g, Sugar 5 g.

Ingredients:

- 453 gramsof 93% lean ground beef

- 1 1/2 teaspoons of kosher salt

- 1 teaspoon of olive oil

- 1/2 large onion, chopped

- 3 cloves of garlic, minced

- 1 28-ounce can of crushed tomatoes

- 2 tablespoons of chopped fresh basil

- Black pepper, to taste

- 3 (8 ounces each) medium zucchinis, sliced 1/8" thick

- 1 1/2 cups of part-skim ricotta

- 1/4 cup of parmesan cheese

- 1 large egg

- 4 cups (16 ounces) of shredded part-skim mozzarella cheese

Instructions:

1. Place the brown meat in a medium saucepan and season with salt. Drain in the colander when cooked to remove any fat.

2. Add the olive oil to the pan and cook for 2 minutes with the garlic and onions. Put the meat back in the pan, then add the tomatoes, basil, salt, and pepper. Simmer for at least 30-40 minutes on the low, covered. The sauce should be thick, so do not add extra water.

3. In the meantime, slice zucchini into 1/8" thick slices, add salt gently and set aside for 10 minutes. When cooked, zucchini has a lot of water, salting it takes a lot of moisture out. Blot excess moisture with a paper towel after 10 minutes.

4. Preheat to medium-high a gas grill or grill pan, and grill 2-3 minutes per side, until slightly browned. To soak up excess moisture, put on paper towels.

5. Preheat oven to 375 degrees Fahrenheit.

6. Combine the ricotta cheese, parmesan cheese, and egg in a medium bowl. Stir well.

7. Spread ½ cup of sauce on the bottom and layer the zucchini to cover in a 9x12 casserole. Spread ½ cup of the mixture of ricotta cheese, then top with 1 cup of mozzarella cheese and repeat the process until all the ingredients are used up. Top the last layer with remaining zucchini and sauce, cover with foil and bake for 30 minutes. Uncover the foil and bake for 20 minutes (to dry the sauce).

8. Let stand before serving for around 5-10 minutes.

20. Lemon Garlic Dump Chicken

(Ready in 50 Minutes, Serve 8, Difficulty: Normal)

Nutrition per Serving:

Calories 255, Protein 36 g, Fat 11 g, Sodium 197mg, Potassium 632mg.

Ingredients:

- 2 teaspoons of minced garlic

- 1/4 cup of olive oil

- 1 tablespoon of parsley flakes

- 2 tablespoons of lemon juice or the juice of 1 whole lemon

- 6 chicken breasts or 8-10 chicken tenders

Instructions:

1. In a 1-gallon freezer bag, put all of the ingredients. I used ½ gallon mason jar with a large mouth to keep the bag upright as I filled it with the chicken and other ingredients.

2. Turn the bag over several times after sealing the bag until everything is mixed and the chicken is well coated. Freeze flat.

3. At the same time, I wanted to make some of these meals to store them in my freezer to be used later. This is my stack of ready-made dump chicken dinners all ready for the freezer!

Option 1—Bake:

Thaw chicken. Pour chicken and marinade into a baking dish, turn chicken to coat. Bake at 350 degrees Fahrenheit (176 Celsius) for 35 minutes.

Option 2—Grill:

Thaw and grill in a cast-iron skillet on the stove, or outside on the barbecue grill, until no longer pink inside.

Option 3—Slow Cooker:

Place the frozen chicken in your slow cooker and cook on low for 6-8 hours (or high for 4-6 hours.)

21. Mushroom-Stuffed Cabbage Rolls

(Ready in 1 Hour and 50 Minutes, Serve 1, Difficulty: Hard)

Nutrition per Serving:

Calories 167, Protein 4.9 g, Carbohydrates 23.7 g, Fat 7.6 g, Cholesterol 0mg, Sodium 218mg.

Ingredients:

- 1 large head cabbage, cored

- 2 tablespoons of olive oil, divided

- 1 medium onion, minced

- ¼ cup of fresh thyme leaves, divided

- 3 cloves of garlic, chopped

- 340 g of finely chopped mushrooms

- ½ cup of raisins

- 1 teaspoon of ground cinnamon

- ¾ cup of roughly chopped walnuts

- 1 teaspoon of sea salt, or to taste, divided

- ½ cup of uncooked brown rice

- 1(16 ounce) can of crushed tomatoes, divided

- Ground black pepper to taste

Instructions:

1. To a boil, put a big pot of lightly salted water. Drop the cabbage into the pot and immerse it completely in the wine. For 10 minutes, cook. Remove from the water and allow for about 10 minutes to cool enough to manage. Carefully pull the leaves off.

2. The oven should be preheated to 350 degrees Fahrenheit (176 degrees Celsius).

3. Heat 1 tablespoon of oil over medium to high heat in a large skillet. Add the onion, 1/3 of the garlic, and the thyme. Cook for about 5 minutes, until the onions are translucent. Add the mushrooms, cinnamon, and raisins and cook for about 3 minutes. Stir in the walnuts and add 1/3 of the sea salt to season. Transfer the mixture to a large bowl and incorporate the rice into a uniform mixture, stirring the stuffing.

4. Grease a baking dish with the remaining olive oil and use a thin layer of tomatoes to line the rim. Sprinkle 1/3 of the thyme, 1/3 of the sea salt, and pepper lightly to taste.

5. Scoop into a cabbage leaf around a heaping tablespoon of stuffing and first fold into the sides, then roll and put in the prepared pan. Repeat with the leaves, and the stuffing left. To close up any broken rolls, use any torn leaves. Top the remaining tomatoes with the rest of the thyme. Season with the remaining pepper and salt.

6. Use aluminum foil or a sheet to cover the baking dish.

7. Bake until tender in the preheated oven, about 45 minutes.

22. Insanely Easy Vegetarian Chili

(Ready in 55 Minutes, Serve 8, Difficulty: Normal)

Nutrition per Serving:

Calories 215, Protein 6.8 g, Carbohydrates 29 g, Fat 3 g, Cholesterol 0mg, Sodium 423.3mg.

Ingredients:

- 1 tablespoon of vegetable oil
- 1 cup of chopped onions
- ¾ cup of chopped carrots
- 3 cloves of garlic, minced
- 1 cup of chopped green bell pepper
- 1 cup of chopped red bell pepper
- ¾ cup of chopped celery
- 1 tablespoon of chili powder
- 1 ½ cups of chopped fresh mushrooms
- 1(28 ounces) can of whole peeled tomatoes with liquid, chopped

- 1(19 ounces) can of kidney beans with liquid

- 1(11 ounces) can of whole kernel corn, undrained

- 1 tablespoon of ground cumin

- 1 ½ teaspoon of dried oregano

- 1 ½ teaspoon of dried basil

Instructions:

1. Heat oil over medium heat in a large saucepan. Sauté the carrots, onions, and garlic until tender. Add the red pepper, green pepper, celery, and chili powder and mix properly. Cook for about 6 minutes, until the vegetables are tender.

2. Add the mushrooms and cook for 4 minutes. Stir in the onions, corn, and kidney beans. Use oregano, and basil to season. Bring to a boil, and reduce to medium heat. Cover and simmer, stirring periodically, for 20 minutes.

Chapter 5: Soups Recipes

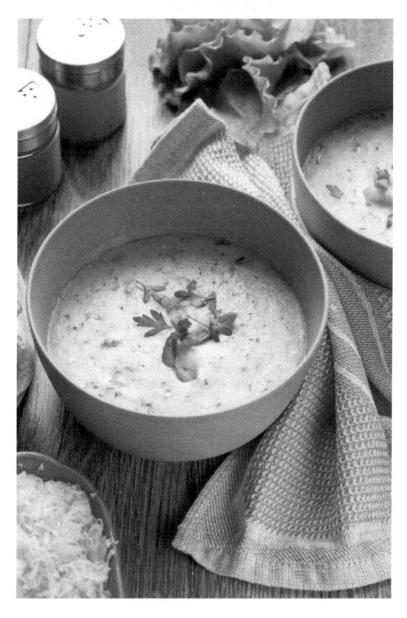

In this chapter, we are going to give you some delicious and mouthwatering recipes on Octavia Soups recipes.

23. Absolutely Ultimate Potato Soup

(Ready in 50 Minutes, Serve 8, Difficulty: Normal)

Nutrition per Serving:

Calories 129, Protein 12.6 g, Carbohydrates 44 g, Fat 41.5 g, Cholesterol 91.2mg, Sodium 879.4mg.

Ingredients:

- 453 g of bacon, chopped

- 2 stalks of celery, diced

- 1 onion, chopped

- 3 cloves of garlic, minced

- 8 potatoes, peeled and cubed

- 4 cups of chicken stock, or enough to cover potatoes

- 3 tablespoons of butter

- ¼ cup of all-purpose flour

- 1 cup of heavy cream

- 1 teaspoon of dried tarragon

- 3 teaspoons of chopped fresh cilantro

- Salt and pepper, to taste

Instructions:

1. Cook the bacon in a Dutch oven over medium heat until done. Take the bacon out of the grill, and set it aside. Drain the bacon fat from all but ¼ cup.

2. In the reserved bacon drippings, cook the celery and onion until the onion is translucent, about 5 minutes. Add the garlic, and proceed to cook for 1-2 minutes. To coat, add the cubed potatoes and toss.

3. Cook for between 3-4 minutes. Place the bacon back in the pan and add more chicken stock to cover the potatoes. Cover and boil until tender, then cook the potatoes.

4. Melt the butter over medium heat in a separate pan. Whisk the flour in. Cook for 1-2 minutes, continuously stirring. Heavy cream, tarragon, and cilantro are whisked in. Bring the cream mixture to a boil, and simmer until it thickens, stirring continuously. Into the potato mixture, stir the cream mixture.

5. Mash about 1/2 of the soup and return to the pan. Adjust the seasonings according to taste.

24. Fresh Asparagus Soup

(Ready in 30 Minutes, Serve 4, Difficulty: Easy)

Nutrition per Serving:

Calories 167, Protein 9.7 g, Carbohydrates 18.7 g, Fat 6.7 g, Cholesterol 15mg, Sodium 966.8mg.

Ingredients:

- 453 g of fresh asparagus

- ¾ cup of chopped onion

- ½ cup of vegetable broth

- 1 tablespoon of butter

- 2 tablespoons of all-purpose flour

- 1 teaspoon of salt

- 1 pinch of ground black pepper

- 1 ¼ cups of vegetable broth

- 1 cup of soy milk

- ½ cup of yogurt

- 1 teaspoon of lemon juice

- ¼ cup of grated parmesan cheese

Instructions:

1. In a saucepan with 1/2 cup vegetable broth, put the asparagus and onion. Bring the broth to a boil, reduce the heat, and let the vegetables cook until tender.

2. For garnish, reserve a few asparagus tips. In an electric mixer, put the remaining vegetable mixture and puree until smooth.

3. In the pan that was used for simmering the asparagus and onions, melt the butter. While the starch, salt, and pepper are sprinkled into the sugar, whisk. Do not let the flour brown. Let the mixture cook for only 2 minutes. Increase the heat and stir the remaining 1 ¼ cup of vegetable broth. When the mixture comes to a boil, begin stirring.

4. In the saucepan, stir the vegetable puree and milk. Whisk the yogurt, followed by the lemon juice, into the mixture. Stir until fully heated, then ladle into bowls. With reserved asparagus tops, garnish. If needed, sprinkle with parmesan cheese.

25. Healing Cabbage Soup

(Ready in 1 Hour and. 15 Minutes, Serve 8, Difficulty: Normal)

Nutrition per Serving:

Calories 228, Protein 1.5 g, Carbohydrates 8.6 g, Fat 5.2 g, Cholesterol 0mg, Sodium 435.9mg.

Ingredients:

- 3 tablespoons of olive oil
- ½ onion, chopped
- 2 cloves of garlic, chopped
- 2 quarts of water
- 4 teaspoons of chicken bouillon granules
- 1 teaspoon of salt, or to taste
- ½ teaspoon of black pepper, or to taste
- ½ head of cabbage, cored and coarsely chopped
- 1(14.5 ounces) can of Italian-style stewed tomatoes, drained and diced

Instructions:

1. Heat olive oil over medium heat in a large stockpot. Stir in the onion and garlic and simmer for about 5 minutes until the onion is clear.

2. Add sugar, bouillon, salt, and pepper and stir. Bring it to a boil, and add the cabbage. Simmer for about 10 minutes before the cabbage wilts.

3. Stir the tomatoes in. Return to the boil and simmer for 15-30 minutes, stirring regularly.

26. Avgolemono

(Ready in 30 Minutes, Serve 4, Difficulty: Easy)

Nutrition per Serving:

Calories 150, Protein 8.4 g, Carbohydrates 21.8 g, Fat 4.2 g, Cholesterol 139.5mg, Sodium 54.6mg.

Ingredients:

- 1 ¾ quart of chicken broth
- ½ cup of uncooked orzo pasta
- 3 eggs
- 1 lemon, juiced
- 1 tablespoon of cold water
- Salt and pepper, to taste

Instructions:

1. In a large saucepan, pour the chicken broth, and bring it to a boil. Stir in the pasta, then simmer for 5 minutes.

2. Add the lemon juice and 1 tablespoon of cold water, then beat the eggs until frothy. Stir the hot chicken stock slowly into a ladleful, then add one or 2 more. Be alert not to scramble through the eggs!

3. Bring this mixture back into the pan, put it off the flame, and stir well. Season with salt and pepper and serve with lemon slices garnished at once. If the eggs have been added, do not let the soup boil, or it will curdle!

27. Chunky Chicken Noodle Soup

(Ready in 25 Minutes, Serve 1, Difficulty: Easy)

Nutrition per Serving:

Calories 210, Protein 8.8 g, Carbohydrates 13.2 g, Fat 1.6 g, Cholesterol 26.5mg, Sodium 1233.5mg.

Ingredients:

- 3 quarts of water

- 1(32 fluid ounces) container of chicken stock

- 8 cubes of chicken bouillon

- 3 skinless, boneless chicken breast halves, cut into 1-inch pieces

- 4 cups of egg noodles

- 1 cup of frozen peas and carrots

- 2 carrots, chopped

- 2 stalks of celery, chopped

- ¼ cup of chopped onion

- 1 teaspoon of salt

- 1 teaspoon of ground black pepper

- ¼ teaspoon of dried basil

- ⅛ teaspoon of crushed bay leaf

- ⅛ teaspoon of dried oregano

Instructions:

1. In a large stockpot, put the water, chicken stock, and chicken bouillon to a boil. Put in the chicken breast, the egg noodles, the peas and vegetables, the sliced carrots, the celery, the onion, the garlic, the black pepper, the basil, the bay leaves, and the oregano.

2. Continue to simmer for 20 minutes, uncovered. Reduce the heat to mild and cook until the chicken in the center is no longer pink and the noodles are soft, 5-10 more minutes.

28. Spaetzle and Chicken Soup

(Ready in 2 hrs. 20 Minutes, Serve 8, and Difficulty: Hard)

Nutrition per Serving:

Calories 126, Protein 36.3 g, Carbohydrates 45.3 g, Fat 25.2 g, Cholesterol 222.7mg, Sodium 648mg.

Ingredients:

- 1(1360 g) of a whole chicken
- 2(14.5 ounces) of cans chicken broth
- 2 medium yellow onions, quartered
- 1 bunch of celery with leaves, cut into pieces
- 1(16 ounces) package of baby carrots
- Salt and ground black pepper, to taste
- ½ teaspoon of garlic salt, or to taste
- 5 eggs
- ½ cup of water
- 1 teaspoon of salt
- 3 cups of all-purpose flour
- ½ teaspoon of parsley flakes

Instructions:

1. Place the chicken and add enough water to cover it in a stockpot. Pour in the chicken broth and add the onions and celery. Add salt, pepper, and garlic salt to the seasoning. Bring it to a boil and simmer for 1 hour or so to get a healthy broth.

2. Remove it to a plate when the chicken is cooked and tender, and let sit until it is cool enough to treat. Strain the broth and discard the onions and celery. Take the broth back to the stockpot. Strip the chicken meat from the bones, slice it or break it into bits, and add it to the oven. Boil the broth and add the carrots.

3. Then stir together the eggs, water, and salt in a medium dish. Add flour gradually until the dough is firm enough for a ball to form. You can need more flour or less. On a flat plate, pat the dough out. Cut slices of dough from the side of the plate with a butter knife until they are around 2-3 inches long. Allow them to fall straight into the broth that is boiling.

4. The soup is ready until the carrots are tender. Sprinkle with flakes of parsley and serve.

Chapter 6: Vegan Recipes

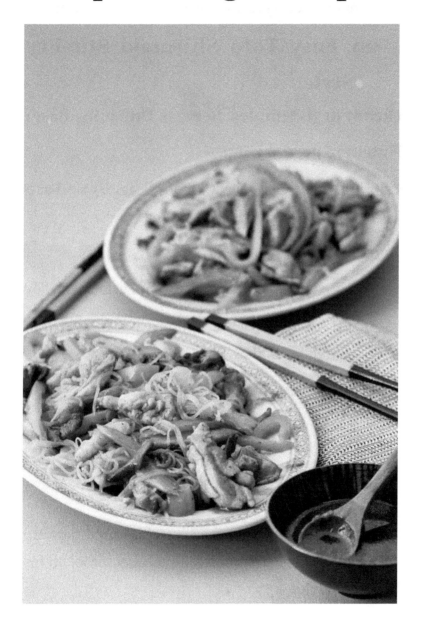

In this chapter we are going to give you some delicious and mouthwatering recipes on Octavia Vegan recipes.

29. Easy Tofu Shirataki Stir-Fry Style

(Ready in 30 Minutes, Serve 6, Difficulty: Easy)

Nutrition per Serving:

Calories 139, Protein 5.7 g, Carbohydrates 29.8 g, Fat 0 g, Cholesterol 0mg, Sodium 628.4mg.

Ingredients:

- 1(16 ounces) package of frozen vegetable medley
- 1(8 ounces) package of angel hair-style tofu Shirataki noodles, or to taste
- ½ teaspoon of minced garlic
- 2 teaspoons of soy sauce, or to taste
- ½ teaspoon of ground ginger, or to taste

Instructions:

1. In the pot, microwave the vegetables until they are thawed and cooked, about 5 minutes. Let it cool off for about 1 minute.

2. Drain and thoroughly rinse the Shirataki noodles and put them in a microwave-safe dish.

3. In the microwave, cook the noodles until mostly heated, around 1 minute.

4. Heat a saucepan and add garlic over medium heat. Cook for around 1 minute before fragrant. Add the fried pasta, soy sauce, mixed vegetables, and ginger. Cook and stir until heated and blended with flavors, 2-3 minutes. Stir in spicy sauce.

30. Vegan Stuffed Peppers with Rice

(Ready in 55 Minutes, Serve 6, Difficulty: Normal)

Nutrition per Serving:

Calories 229, Protein 19.2 g, Carbohydrates 51.8 g, Fat 2.6 g, Cholesterol 0mg, Sodium 1116.1mg.

Ingredients:

- 4 red bell peppers, tops, and seeds removed

- Salt, to taste

- 1 cup of vegan "ground beef," frozen (such as Beyond Meat®)

- 1 cup of diced onion

- 1 cup of diced tomatoes

- 1(14 ounces) can of vegetable broth, divided

- 1 teaspoon of garlic powder

- 1 teaspoon of chili powder

- ½ teaspoon of ground black pepper

- 1 cup of water

- 1(8 ounces) package of Spanish rice mix

- 1 cup of black beans, rinsed and drained

- 1 cup of corn, drained

- 1 tablespoon of nutritional yeast (optional)

- 4 ounces of tomato sauce

Instructions:

1. To a simmer, put a big pot of water. Add the bell peppers and cook for 8-10 minutes, until tender. Drain and sprinkle salt on the inside. Place 10 minutes free.

2. The oven should be preheated to 350 degrees Fahrenheit (176 degrees Celsius). Line an aluminum foil baking tray with it.

3. In a large skillet over medium-high heat, mix vegan ground beef, onion, diced tomatoes, 2/3 cup broth, garlic powder, chili powder, black pepper, and salt bring to a high boil. Cook until all but 1/3 cup of liquid has steamed off or been consumed, 5-10 minutes, stirring periodically. Remove from the heat.

4. In a saucepan, mix water, 1 cup broth, and Spanish rice packet over medium heat. Bring to a boil, simmer, and cook for 8 minutes. Minimize pressure. Add the corn and black beans and mix to blend. Add the mixture of ground beef with adequate liquid to keep the rice stuffing moist. Add and stir in the nutritional yeast until well mixed.

5. Drain the peppers with any extra water. Using a spoon to stuff with rice mixture, packing securely to fill off. In the prepared baking pan, put the stuffed peppers and spoon the extra rice mixture around them. Pour the tomato sauce over the rice and peppers with aluminum foil shell.

6. Bake for 20 minutes in the preheated oven. Remove the foil and bake for an extra 10 minutes, uncovered. Until eating, let the peppers rest for 5 minutes.

31. Pressure Cooker Sambar (Indian Lentil Curry)

(Ready in 30 Minutes, Serve 4, Difficulty: Easy)

Nutrition per Serving:

Calories 238, Protein 14.8 g, Carbohydrates 41 g, Fat 2.4 g, Cholesterol 0mg, Sodium 47.2mg.

Ingredients:

- 6 ½ cups of water, divided
- 1 cup of yellow lentils
- 1 cup of chopped eggplant
- 1 teaspoon of turmeric powder
- Salt, to taste
- 1 tablespoon of tamarind paste
- 2 teaspoons of ground red Chile powder
- 1 teaspoon of vegetable oil, or as needed
- 1 whole dried-red Chile
- 4 curry leaves, or more to taste
- 1 teaspoon of whole cumin seeds
- 1 teaspoon of mustard seeds

- 1 pinch of asafoetida powder

Instructions:

1. In a pressure cooker, mix 4 cups of water, lentils, eggplant, turmeric, and salt. Cover the cooker safely and position the pressure regulator over the vent as instructed by the manufacturer. Heat until steam, about 10 minutes, exits in a constant flow and makes a whistling sound. Switch the temperature until the controller is rocking softly. Cook and exit from the heat for 3 minutes. As per the manufacturer's instructions, let the pressure release naturally for 5-10 minutes. Unlock the lid and remove it.

2. Add to the pressure cooker the remaining 2 1/2 cups of water, tamarind paste, and chili powder. Cover the cooker safely and position the pressure regulator over the vent as instructed by the manufacturer. Heat until steam, about 10 minutes, exits in a constant flow and makes a whistling sound. Remove from heat. As per the manufacturer's instructions, let the pressure release naturally for 5-10 minutes. Unlock the lid and remove it.

3. In a shallow saucepan, mix the oil, dried chili, curry leaves, cumin seeds, mustard seeds, and asafoetida powder over low heat. Cook for about 1 minute before the spices begin to sputter a little. Move the spice mixture and the lentils to the pressure cooker. Season with salt.

32. Homemade Vegetable Sushi

(Ready in1 Hour and 10 Minutes, Serve 18, Difficulty: Hard)

Nutrition per Serving:

Calories 216, Protein 1.1 g, Carbohydrates 10.5 g, Fat 1.7 g, Cholesterol 0mg, Sodium 4.1mg

Ingredients:

- 1 cup of sushi rice
- 1 cup of water
- 3 sheets sushi nori (dry seaweed)
- ⅓ cup of rice vinegar
- 1 small cucumber, cut into matchstick-size pieces
- 1 carrot, cut into matchstick-size pieces
- 1 avocado, sliced

Instructions:

1. In cool water, clean the sushi rice and drain. Put the rice and 1 cup of water in a rice cooker. Seal and pick the setting as instructed by the manufacturer, cook

until tender, around 15 minutes. With a fork, fluff, and let sit for 10 minutes.

2. On the sugar, add the rice vinegar and toss to coat. Let it cool absolutely for about thirty minutes.

3. Cover the plastic wrap with a bamboo sushi mat and put it on a cutting board. On the covered sushi mat, put a sheet of nori and cover it with cooled rice.

4. Spread out on top of 1/3 of the cucumber, carrot, and avocado, placing them around the boards bottom third. To help roll the nori up, use the sushi mat. Repeat with the nori, corn, and vegetables left. To cut each roll into six similar pieces, use a sharp knife.

33. Easy Creamy Vegan Mushroom Risotto

(Ready in 45 Minutes, Serve 6, Difficulty: Normal)

Nutrition per Serving:

Calories 327, Protein 12.4 g, Carbohydrates 65.7 g, Fat 1.9 g, Cholesterol 0mg, Sodium 921.2mg.

Ingredients:

- 1 onion, chopped

- 2 cloves of garlic, minced

- 2 teaspoons of Provence herb

- 2 ¼ cups of vegetable broth, or as needed, divided

- 2 cups of white mushrooms, sliced

- ½ cup of chopped leek

- 1 cup of Arborio rice

- 1 cup of soy milk

- 1 tablespoon of white wine vinegar

- 1 cup of frozen peas

- 2 tablespoons of lemon juice

- 2 tablespoons of nutritional yeast

- 1 teaspoon of salt

- ½ teaspoon of ground black pepper

Instructions:

1. Over a medium-high flame, heat a large saucepan. Cook the tomato, ginger, and Provence herbs. Should the mixture be too dry, add some vegetable broth to the mixture. Add the mushrooms and leeks and cook for 3-4 minutes, until heated.

2. Pour the leftover rice and vegetable broth into the mushroom mixture. Add vinegar and soy milk. Let it boil for 15-20 minutes before the liquid is absorbed, stirring periodically.

3. Stir in the rice mixture with the peas, lemon juice, and nutritional yeast. Cook until the peas, about 3 minutes, are cooked through. Turn off the heat, add salt and pepper, to season.

34. Easy, Healthy Falafel

(Ready in 30 Minutes, Serve 1, Difficulty: Normal)

Nutrition per Serving:

Calories 246, Protein 1.6 g, Carbohydrates 7.8 g, Fat 1 g, Cholesterol 0mg, Sodium 106.9mg.

Ingredients:

- 1(14 ounces) can of chickpeas

- 1 onion, chopped

- 3 tablespoons of chopped flat, leaf parsley, or to taste

- 2 teaspoons of olive oil

- 2 cloves of garlic, chopped, or to taste

- 1 teaspoon of coriander

- 1 teaspoon of cumin

- Salt and pepper, to taste

- 2 tablespoons of all-purpose flour

- ½ teaspoon of baking powder

Instructions:

1. The oven should be preheated to 400 degrees Fahrenheit (204 degrees Celsius).

2. In the bowl of a food processor, combine the chickpeas, cabbage, parsley, oil, garlic, cilantro, and salt, and pepper, pulse until everything is combined. Add flour and baking powder and pulse until the mixture begins to bind together and forms a ball and if necessary, scrape the sides of the bowl.

3. To extract even volumes of the mixture, use two dessert spoons and form them into 15 small patties. On a baking sheet, put the patties.

4. Bake for 25-30 minutes in the preheated oven until golden brown, turning the falafel over carefully after 10 minutes.

Chapter 7: Meat Dishes

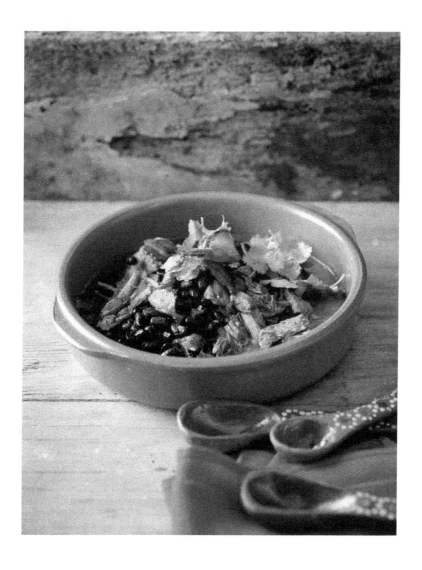

In this chapter, we are going to give you some delicious and mouthwatering recipes on Lean & Green Meat Dishes recipes.

35. Meat in its Juices

(Ready in 55 Minutes, Serve 6, Difficulty: Normal)

Nutrition per Serving:

Calories 337, Protein 29.2 g, Carbohydrates 27.5 g, Fat 16.3 g, Cholesterol 57.8mg, Sodium 860.2mg.

Ingredients:

- 6 slices of bacon

- 4 fresh tomatillos, husks removed

- 3 serrano Chile peppers, seeded and chopped

- 1 clove of garlic, peeled

- 3 cups of water

- 907 g of flank steak, cut into 1/2-inch squares

- 1 cube of chicken bouillon

- 2(15.5 ounces) cans of pinto beans

- ½ onion, chopped

- 6 tablespoons of chopped fresh cilantro

- Ground black pepper, to taste

- 1 lime, cut into 6 wedges

Instructions:

1. Over medium-high heat, cook the bacon in a large deep skillet until crispy, around 10 minutes. Drain it on a tray lined with paper towels. Crumble and Set aside the bacon.

2. In a small saucepan over medium-high heat, add the tomatillos, serrano peppers, garlic, and water, bring to a boil, cover, and simmer for 10 minutes. Take the pan out of the heat and allow it to cool

3. To a blender, move the contents and blend until smooth. Only put aside. If you like, you can skip the simmering phase and mix all the raw ingredients with a few browned flank steak bits.

4. Over medium-high heat, place the non-stick skillet and cook the flank steak in the hot skillet until fully browned. Pour a combination of tomatillo over the beef and bring to a boil. In the mixture, stir the chicken bouillon and reduce the heat to mild. Cover the skillet and cook for at least 30 minutes and up to 1 hour, until tender.

5. Meanwhile, in a saucepan, heat the pinto beans over medium heat until warm, reduce the heat to a minimum, and remain warm until necessary. In the flank steak mixture, stir the bacon and pinto beans and split the mixture between 6 cups. Garnish each with a slice of onion, coriander, black pepper, and lime.

36. Classic and Simple Meat Lasagna

(Ready in 1 Hour and 35 Minutes, Serve 8, Difficulty: Hard)

Nutrition per Serving:

Calories 250, Protein 35.6 g, Carbohydrates 47.1 g, Fat 19.3 g, Cholesterol 114.5mg, Sodium 999mg.

Ingredients:

- 12 whole wheat lasagna noodles

- 453 g of lean ground beef

- 2 cloves of garlic, chopped

- ½ teaspoon of garlic powder

- 1 teaspoon of dried oregano, or to taste

- Salt and ground black pepper, to taste

- 1(16 ounces) package of cottage cheese

- 2 eggs

- ½ cup of shredded parmesan cheese

- 1 ½ (25 ounces) jars of tomato-basil pasta sauce

- 2 cups of shredded mozzarella cheese

Instructions:

1. Preheat the oven to 350 degrees Fahrenheit (176 degrees Celsius).

2. Fill a large pot with thinly salted water and bring it over high heat to a rolling boil. When the water has cooked, add a few lasagna noodles at a time and return to the boil.

3. Cook the uncovered pasta, stirring regularly, until the pasta is thoroughly cooked but still strong to the bite, around 10 minutes. Place the noodles on a tray.

4. Put the ground beef in a medium-hot saucepan and Combine the garlic, garlic powder, oregano, salt, and black pepper to the saucepan. Cook the meat until it's no longer yellow, about 10 minutes, and cut it into small chunks as it cooks. Drain the excess grease.

5. Mix the cottage cheese, eggs, and Parmesan cheese in a bowl until completely mixed.

6. In a 9x13-inch baking pan, put four noodles side by side on the bottom, top with a layer of tomato-basil sauce, a layer of ground beef mixture, and a layer of cottage cheese mixture. Repeat the layers, finish with a layer of sauce, and scatter the mozzarella cheese on top. In aluminum foil, protect the bowl.

7. Bake for about 30 minutes in the preheated oven until the casserole is bubbling and the cheese has melted. Remove the foil and bake for about 10 more minutes before the cheese has started to brown. Allow it to stand before serving for at least 10 minutes.

37. Restaurant-Style Taco Meat Seasoning

(Ready in 40 Minutes, Serve 10, Difficulty: Normal)

Nutrition per Serving:

Calories 316, Protein 10.6 g, Carbohydrates 2.1 g, Fat 12.4 g, Cholesterol 43.6mg, Sodium 212.1mg.

Ingredients:

- 1 ½ tablespoon of corn flour

- 4 ½ teaspoons of chili powder

- ½ teaspoon of onion powder

- ½ teaspoon of garlic powder

- ½ teaspoon of seasoned salt

- ½ teaspoon of paprika

- ¼ teaspoon of cumin

- ½ teaspoon of garlic salt

- ¼ teaspoon of sugar

- 1 teaspoon of dried minced onion

- ½ teaspoon of beef bouillon granules

- ¼ teaspoon of ground red pepper

- 604 g lean of ground chuck

- 1 cup of water

Instructions:

1. Preheat the oven to 350 degrees Fahrenheit (176 degrees Celsius).

2. Pour a large pot with thinly salted water and bring it to a rolling boil over high heat. Add a few lasagna

noodles after the water has cooked, then return to the boil.

3. Cook the uncovered pasta for about 10 minutes, occasionally stirring, until the pasta is thoroughly cooked but still firm to the bite. Place it on a tray with the noodles.

4. In a medium-hot saucepan, put the ground beef and add the garlic, garlic powder, oregano, salt, and black pepper to the saucepan. Cook the meat for about 10 minutes, until it's no longer pink, then cut it into small chunks as it cooks. Drain the grease from the excess.

5. In a bowl, combine the cottage cheese, eggs, and parmesan cheese until thoroughly combined.

6. Place four noodles side by side in a 9x13-inch baking pan on the bottom, top with a layer of tomato-basil sauce, a layer of ground beef mixture, and a cottage layer cheese mixture. Repeat the layers, combine a layer of sauce to the finish, and spread the mozzarella cheese on top. Cover the bowl with aluminum foil.

7. Bake in the preheated oven for about 30 minutes until the casserole is bubbling and the cheese has melted. Before the cheese begins to brown, cut the foil and bake for about ten more minutes. Allow it to stand for at least 10 minutes before serving.

38. Meat-Lover's Slow Cooker Spaghetti Sauce

(Ready in 8 Hour and 40 Minutes, Serve 8, and Difficulty: Normal)

Nutrition per Serving:

Calories 264, Protein 15 g, Carbohydrates 18.8 g, Fat 14.8 g, Cholesterol 45.2mg, Sodium 1025.1mg.

Ingredients:

- 2 tablespoons of olive oil
- 2 small onions, chopped
- 113 g of bulk Italian sausage
- 453 g of ground beef
- 1 teaspoon of dried Italian herb seasoning
- 1 teaspoon of garlic powder
- ½ teaspoon of dried marjoram
- 1(29 ounces) can of tomato sauce
- 1(6 ounces) can of tomato paste
- 1(14.5 ounces) can of Italian-style diced tomatoes

- 1(14.5 ounces) can of Italian-style stewed tomatoes

- ¼ teaspoon of dried thyme leaves

- ¼ teaspoon of dried basil

- ½ teaspoon of dried oregano

- 2 teaspoons of garlic powder

- 1 tablespoon of white sugar

Instructions:

1. Heat the olive oil over medium heat in a pan, cook and stir in the onions and the Italian sausage until browned, about 10 minutes.

2. To a slow cooker, pass the sausage and onions. Cook the ground beef, the Italian seasoning, one teaspoon of garlic powder, and marjoram in the same skillet and mix, breaking the meat as it cooks until the meat is browned, about 10 minutes. Through the slow cooker, pass the ground beef.

3. Stir in the tomato sauce, the tomato paste, the sliced tomatoes, the stewed tomatoes, the thyme, the basil, the oregano, and the garlic powder for 2 teaspoons. Place the cooker on the low side and steam the sauce

for 8 hours. Stir in the sugar roughly 15 minutes before serving. Serve it hot.

39. Good New Orleans Creole Gumbo

(Ready in 3 Hours and 40 Minutes, Serve 20, and Difficulty: Normal)

Nutrition per Serving:

Calories 283, Protein 20.9 g, Carbohydrates 12.1 g, Fat 16.6 g, Cholesterol 142.6mg, Sodium 853.1mg.

Ingredients:

- 1 cup of all-purpose flour

- ¾ cup of bacon drippings

- 1 cup of coarsely chopped celery

- 1 large onion, coarsely chopped

- 1 large green bell pepper, coarsely chopped

- 2 cloves of garlic, minced

- 453 g of Andouille sausage, sliced

- 3 quarts of water

- 6 cubes of beef bouillon

- 1 tablespoon of white sugar

- Salt, to taste

- 2 tablespoons of hot pepper sauce (such as Tabasco®), or to taste

- ½ teaspoon of Cajun seasoning blend (such as Tony Chachere's®), or to taste

- 4 bay leaves

- ½ teaspoon of dried thyme leaves

- 1(14.5 ounces) can of stewed tomatoes

- 1(6 ounces) can of tomato sauce

- 2 teaspoons of gumbo file powder

- 2 tablespoons of bacon drippings

- 2(10 ounces) packages of frozen cut okra, thawed

- 2 tablespoons of distilled white vinegar

- 453 g of lump crabmeat

- 1360 g of uncooked medium shrimp, peeled and deveined

- 2 tablespoons of Worcestershire sauce

- 2 teaspoons of gumbo file powder

Instructions:

1. Create a roux to form a smooth mixture by whisking the flour and 3/4 cup bacon drippings together in a large, heavy saucepan over medium-low heat. Cook the roux until it turns a deep mahogany brown color, whisking vigorously.

2. It will take 20 to 30 minutes, closely watch the heat and continuously whisk or roux can fire. Remove from the heat and whisk until the mixture has finished heating.

3. In the working bowl of a food processor, put the celery, onion, green bell pepper, garlic, and pulse until the vegetables are very finely chopped. In the roux, stir the onions, and pour in the sausage. Bring the mixture to a boil over medium-low heat and cook for 10-15 minutes until the vegetables are tender. Remove and set aside from the heat.

4. In a big Dutch oven or soup pot, put the water and beef bouillon cubes to a boil. Stir and whisk the roux mixture into the hot water until the bouillon cubes dissolve. Mix the cinnamon, salt, hot pepper sauce, Cajun spices, bay leaves, thyme, stewed tomatoes, and tomato sauce and lower the heat to a simmer. Simmer the broth over low heat for 1 hour, blend at the 45-minute stage with 2 teaspoons of file gumbo powder.

5. Meanwhile, in a pan, melt 2 teaspoons of bacon drippings and cook the okra over medium heat for 15 minutes with the vinegar, scrape the okra with the slotted spoon whisk in the gumbo. Mix in the crabmeat, shrimp, and Worcestershire sauce, and simmer for another 45 minutes before the flavors have merged. Stir in 2 more teaspoons of file gumbo powder just before serving.

40. Chef John's Italian Meatballs

(Ready in 2 Hours and 15 Minutes, Serve 30, and Difficulty: Hard)

Nutrition per Serving:

Calories 282, Protein 6.2 g, Carbohydrates 1.7 g, Fat 5.5 g, Cholesterol 32.3mg, Sodium 192.1mg.

Ingredients:

- ⅓ cup of plain bread crumbs

- ½ cup of milk

- 2 tablespoons of olive oil

- 1 onion, diced

- 453 g of ground beef

- 453 g of ground pork

- 2 eggs

- ¼ bunch of fresh parsley, chopped

- 3 cloves of garlic, crushed

- 2 teaspoons of salt

- 1 teaspoon of ground black pepper

- ½ teaspoon of red pepper flakes

- 1 teaspoon of dried Italian herb seasoning

- 2 tablespoons of grated parmesan cheese

Instructions:

1. Using foil to protect a baking sheet and brush loosely with cooking spray.

2. Soak the bread crumbs in milk for 20 minutes in a small bowl.

3. Heat olive oil over low heat in a skillet. Cook and mix the onions in hot oil for around 20 minutes, until translucent.

4. In a large tub, combine the beef and pork. Stir in the meat mixture with the rubber spatula once combined: onions, bread crumb mixture, eggs, parsley, garlic, cinnamon, black pepper, red pepper flakes, Italian herb seasoning, and parmesan cheese. Cover for about 1 hour and refrigerate.

5. Preheat the oven to 425 degrees Fahrenheit (218 degrees Celsius).

6. Shape the meat mixture into balls about 1 1/2 inches in diameter using wet hands. Arrange it on a ready baking dish.

7. In the preheated oven, bake for 15-20 minutes until browned and cooked through.

Chapter 8: Salad Recipes

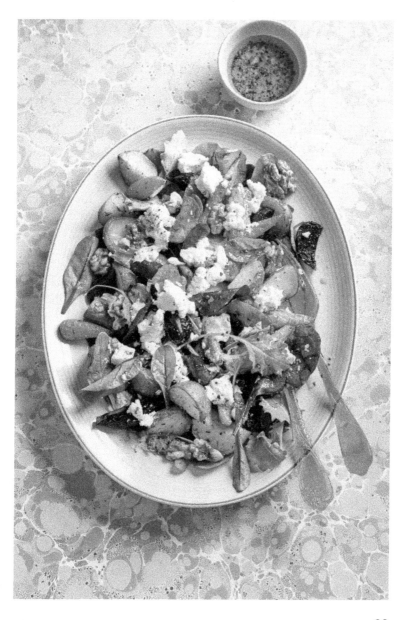

In this chapter we are going to give you some delicious and mouthwatering recipes on Lean & Green Salad recipes.

41. Warm Green Bean and Potato Salad with Goat Cheese

(Ready in 40 Minutes, Serve 8, Difficulty: Normal)

Nutrition per Serving:

Calories 252, Protein 9.2 g, Carbohydrates 28.6 g, Fat 9.6 g, Cholesterol 22.4mg, Sodium 404.1mg.

Ingredients:

- 907 g of red potatoes, cut into bite-size pieces

- 1 serving olive oil cooking spray

- 226 g of frozen French-style green beans, thawed

- 1 cup of chopped red onion

- 4 cloves of garlic, minced

- ½ cup of reduced-fat balsamic vinaigrette dressing

- 1 cup of jarred roasted red peppers, drained and chopped

- ¼ cup of chopped fresh basil

- 1(8 ounces) package of goat cheese, crumbled

Instructions:

1. Place the potatoes and cover them with salted water in a big jar. Bring over high heat to a boil, reduce heat to medium-low, cover and simmer for 8-10 minutes until tender.

2. Drain and allow to dry for 1 minute or 2 while steaming. Place the potatoes in a big bowl.

3. Heat a large skillet over medium-high heat, cooking spray oil. Cook and mix the green beans and onion for about 5 minutes, until tender. Add the garlic, cook, and stir until the garlic is fragrant, about an additional 1 minute.

4. Move the mixture of green beans to the potatoes in a large dish. Lightly toss in the roasted red peppers, balsamic vinaigrette, and basil. Stir in the cheese for the goats.

42. Warm Bok Choy, Beet and Feta Salad

(Ready in 40 Minutes, Serve 3, Difficulty: Normal)

Nutrition per Serving:

Calories 212, Protein 5.5 g, Carbohydrates 12.5 g, Fat 16.5 g, Cholesterol 20.2mg, Sodium 333.7mg.

Ingredients:

- 4 small beets, trimmed, leaving 1 inch of stems Added

- 4 cloves of garlic, chopped, divided

- 1 teaspoon of olive oil

- 3 heads of baby bok Choy, chopped

- 2 tablespoons of peanut oil

- 1 ½ teaspoon of butter

- ⅓ cup of crumbled feta cheese

Instructions:

1. Preheat the oven to 425 degrees Fahrenheit (218 degrees Celsius). On a piece of heavy aluminum foil,

put the beets, ¼ of the chopped garlic, and the olive oil, and fold the foil into a sealed packet around the beets.

2. Roast the beets in the preheated oven for 40 minutes to 1 hour before they are easily pierced with a fork.

3. Only let the beets cool so they can be treated, then rub to loosen the skin with a paper towel. Set aside to slice into ½-inch squares.

4. In a heavy skillet over medium-high pressure, heat the peanut oil and butter. Cook and stir together Bok Choy and the remaining garlic until bok Choy, about 5 minutes, is slightly softened but still crunchy. Stir in the beets and feta, and remove from the heat. Serve it hot.

43. Arugula Salad with Bacon and Butternut Squash

(Ready in 40 Minutes, Serve 1, Difficulty: Normal)

Nutrition per Serving:

Calories, 211 Protein 13.1 g, Carbohydrates 10.3 g, Fat 14.1 g, Cholesterol 32.3mg, Sodium 368mg.

Ingredients:

- 1 slice of bacon, cut into small pieces
- 2 mushrooms, sliced, or to taste
- ¼ cup of cooked butternut squash cubes
- 2 cups of arugula
- 1-ounce of crumbled goat cheese
- 1 teaspoon of pine nuts
- ¼ teaspoon of cracked black pepper, or to taste

Instructions:

1. Cook the bacon in a skillet over medium-high heat for 2 to 3 minutes, before some of the Fat returns to the pan. Add the mushrooms, cook and stir together for about 5 minutes, until the mushrooms are tender.

2. In the bacon mixture, stir squash cubes and continue cooking until the squash is hot and the bacon is crisp, 3-5 minutes more.

3. Place the arugula in a bowl and cover it with a mixture of bacon, mushroom, and squash. Sprinkle on top of the salad with goat cheese and top with pine nuts. Use crushed black pepper to sprinkle.

44. Roasted Lettuce, Radicchio, and Endive

(Ready in 40 Minutes, Serve 6, Difficulty: Normal)

Nutrition per Serving:

Calories 192, Protein 6.3 g, Carbohydrates 16.7 g, Fat 12.9 g, Cholesterol 2.6mg, Sodium 1108.6mg.

Ingredients:

- 2 heads of radicchio, halved lengthwise

- 2 heads of Belgian endive, halved lengthwise

- 1 head of chicory (curly endive), halved lengthwise

- 1 head of romaine lettuce, halved lengthwise

- 3 tablespoons of olive oil, divided

- ¾ cup of pitted Greek olives

- ½ cup of capers

- 1 tablespoon of dried oregano

- 1 ½ teaspoon of ground thyme

- 1 teaspoon of salt

- 1 teaspoon of ground black pepper

- 1 teaspoon of ground dried Chile pepper (Optional)

- 2 tablespoons of grated Romano cheese (Optional)

Instructions:

1. Preheat the oven to 375 degrees Fahrenheit (190 degrees Celsius). Line a parchment paper baking bowl.

2. On the baking sheet, put the radicchio, chicory, Belgian endive, and Romaine lettuce halves in a single layer. Drizzle the end of 2 tablespoons of olive oil.

3. Combine the olives in a small bowl and the capers.

4. To produce the spice mixture, blend the oregano, salt, black pepper, thyme, and chili pepper in a small dish.

5. Using your fingers to stuff the inner leaves with olives, capers, and seasoning mixture. To avoid stuffing from coming out, wrap the halves together with kitchen string. Drizzle on top of the remaining one tablespoon of olive oil.

6. Bake in a preheated oven for 10-15 minutes, until crispy and wilted. Cut the kitchen string off and sprinkle on top of Romano cheese before serving.

45. Warm Thai Kale Salad

(Ready in 40 Minutes, Serve 4, Difficulty: Normal)

Nutrition per Serving:

Calories 176, Protein 5.1 g, Carbohydrates 15 g, Fat 12.1 g, Cholesterol 0mg, Sodium 321.6mg.

Ingredients:

- 2 tablespoons of olive oil

- ½ red onion, thinly sliced

- 5 cloves of garlic, minced

- 1 tablespoon of minced fresh ginger root

- 2 teaspoons of red pepper flakes

- 4 carrots, thinly sliced

- 3 stalks of celery, thinly sliced

- 8 leaves of kale, stemmed and torn into pieces

- 5 sprigs of fresh cilantro, roughly chopped

- 1 lime, juiced

- 2 teaspoons of fish sauce

- ½ teaspoon of lime zest, or to taste

- 1 small cucumber, cut into matchstick-size pieces (Optional)

- ¼ cup of roasted peanuts (Optional)

- 4 sprigs of fresh mint, roughly chopped (Optional)

Instructions:

1. Over medium, prepare, heat a heavy-bottom skillet, add olive oil and swirl in the skillet. Cook and mix the onion in the hot oil for 3 to 4 minutes, until softened.

2. Combine the flakes of garlic, ginger, and red pepper, cook and stir until slightly browned and fragrant with the garlic and ginger, about 1 minute.

3. Stir in the onion mixture with the carrots and celery, cook and stir for 1 minute. Cook and mix until the kale is mildly wilted, about 45 seconds, and add the kale and cilantro. Stir in the kale mixture, lime juice, fish sauce, and lime zest until the kale is evenly covered in the lime juice.

4. Serve the cucumber, popcorn, mint, and kale salad.

46. Maple Cannellini Bean Salad with Baby Broccoli and Butternut Squash

(Ready in 40 Minutes, Serve 8, Difficulty: Normal)

Nutrition per Serving:

Calories 283, Protein 6 g, Carbohydrates 23.8 g, Fat 7 g, Cholesterol 3.7mg, Sodium 323.2mg.

Ingredients:

- 2(15 ounces) cans of cannellini beans, drained and rinsed
- 1 tablespoon of olive oil
- 1 red onion, chopped
- 1 tablespoon of maple syrup
- 1 tablespoon of olive oil
- 1 cup of peeled, seeded, and diced butternut squash
- 1 tablespoon of maple syrup
- 1 tablespoon of olive oil
- 1 cup of chopped baby broccoli

- ¼ cup of chicken stock

- 1 tablespoon of maple syrup

- ½ teaspoon of dried thyme leaves

- 3 slices of bacon, cooked and crumbled

Instructions:

1. Heat the cannellini beans in a saucepan over low heat.

2. Over medium heat, heat one tablespoon of olive oil in a skillet. Add the red onion, cook and stir until the onion is tender and translucent about 5 minutes. Add one tablespoon of maple syrup, reduce heat to medium-low, cook and stir until very tender and dark brown, about 15 more minutes. Remove from the pan and stir in the beans.

3. Heat one additional tablespoon of olive oil over medium heat in a skillet. Add the butternut squash, cook and stir for about 8 minutes, until tender.

4. Add 1 tablespoon of maple syrup and simmer for about 5 minutes, stirring to coat. Remove the bean mixture from the skillet and add the squash.

5. Over medium heat, heat the remaining one tablespoon of olive oil in a skillet. Add the baby broccoli, cook and stir for about 7 minutes, until tender and bright green. Combine the bean mixture with the broccoli.

6. Pour the chicken stock into the bean mixture, raise the heat to medium-low, and add 1 tablespoon of the remaining maple syrup and thyme to the mixture. Carry to a boil and cook until thoroughly cooked, stirring to combine gently before serving, top with crumbled bacon.

Chapter 9: Dessert Recipes

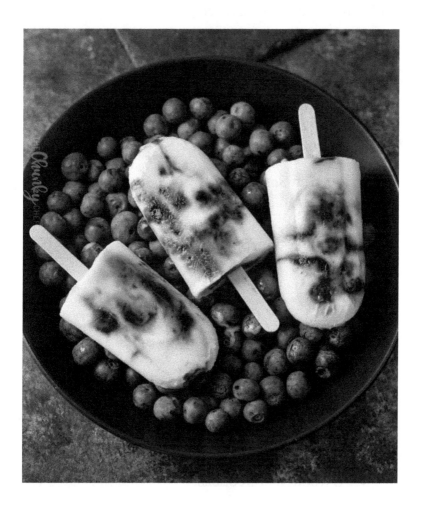

In this chapter, we are going to give you some delicious and mouthwatering recipes

On Lean & Green Dessert recipes.

47. Frozen Blueberry Yogurt Pops

(Ready in 2 Hours and 5 Minutes, Serve 8, and Difficulty: Easy)

Nutrition per Serving:

Calories 237, Protein 0.9 g, Carbohydrates 8.4 g, Fat 0 g, Cholesterol 0.5mg, Sodium 15.3mg.

Ingredients:

- 1 cup of Ocean Spray® Blueberry Juice Cocktail

- 1 cup of Ocean Spray® Fresh Blueberries, cleaned and rinsed

- 1(6 ounces) container of fat-free vanilla yogurt

- 8 wooden craft sticks

Instructions:

1. Combine the blender with all the ingredients. Cover and blend for 15-20 seconds at higher speed, or until smooth.

2. Pour in 8 pop molds that are frozen (2.5 ounces to 3 ounces each). Cover, insert art sticks, and freeze until fully firm or for 2 hours.

3. To serve, dip the exterior of the molds to loosen them in warm water.

48. Cinnamon Gelatin Salad

(Ready in 3 hours and 5 Minutes, Serve 4, and Difficulty: Normal)

Nutrition per Serving:

Calories 165, Protein 2 g, Carbohydrates 40.5 g 1, Fat 0 g, Cholesterol 0mg, Sodium 85.3mg.

Ingredients:

- 1(3 ounces) package of raspberry-flavored Jell-O® Mix

- 1 cup of boiling water

- 1(2.25 ounces) package of cinnamon red-hot candies

- 1 cup of applesauce

Instructions:

1. Mix the gelatin and the hot water in a shallow serving bowl before the gelatin is fully dissolved. Stir in the cinnamon sweets until they are melted, then add in the applesauce. Chill until set, about 3 hours.

49. Almond Ice

(Ready in 4 Hours and 15 Minutes, Serve 12, and Difficulty: Normal)

Nutrition per Serving:

Calories 71, Protein 1.7 g, Carbohydrates 16 g, Fat 0.1 g, Cholesterol 0mg, Sodium 5mg.

Ingredients:

- 5(.25 ounces) envelopes of unflavored gelatin
- 2 ¼ cups of boiling water
- 4 teaspoons of almond extract
- 4 cups of cold water
- 1 ⅓ cup of white sugar
- 1 cup of fresh strawberries, halved
- 1 cup of seedless grapes
- 1 cup cubed cantaloupe

Instructions:

1. In 1 cup of cold water, soften the gelatin. Add 2 ¼ cups of boiling sugar and water. Stir until it dissolves thoroughly. Add 3 cups cold water and the almond extract. Mix thoroughly.

2. In a 9x13-inch pan, pour the gelatin blend and refrigerate for at least 4 hours. Cut into squares of 1 inch and serve with fruits in a bowl.

50. Cranberry Apple Gelatin Mold

(Ready in 8 Hours 20 Minutes, Serve 12, Difficulty: Normal)

Nutrition per Serving:

Calories 180, Protein 3.4 g, Carbohydrates 36.7 g, Fat 3.3 g, Cholesterol 0.3mg, Sodium 121.7mg.

Ingredients:

- 1(16 ounces) can of whole cranberry sauce

- 1 cup of water

- 2(3 ounces) packages of raspberry-flavored Jell-O® Mix

- ¼ teaspoon of salt

- 2 apples, cored and diced with peel

- 2 oranges, peeled, sectioned, and chopped

- ½ cup of chopped walnuts

- 1 cup of lemon yogurt

Instructions:

1. Combine the cranberry sauce and water in a saucepan over medium heat. Heat the sauce until it melts. Stir gelatin until it dissolves. Remove from the heat. Apples, grapes, walnuts, and yogurt are blended in.

2. Pour the mixture into a fancy mold of gelatin or a nice bowl, and cool overnight. Dip briefly in hot water to serve, then invert onto a baking bowl.

Conclusion

The acquisition of new eating habits and the inclusion of physical activity are essential in weight loss and therefore to lead a healthier life. These new practices can help you keep the weight off over time. In addition to improving your health, maintaining the weight you have lost will also greatly improve your life in many ways.

In this case, the Lean & Green diet is a balanced diet to help you lose weight and keep it off. The meals in this diet are designed to be lower in fat, cholesterol, and carbohydrates. This is achieved with fuelings, foods designed to be purposefully low in calories and carbohydrates, and with the right amount of high-quality soy or whey protein.

The "Lean & Green" diet combines meals and a nutritious snack, such as a serving of fruit or a small snack, once the plan is completed, aimed at those who want a higher caloric intake or simply to maintain their ideal weight.

Additionally, low-intensity physical activity for at least 30 minutes is recommended to obtain better results, since physical exercise is the best way to reduce the calories ingested. It should not be forgotten that any weight loss diet loses its intention if it is not combined with moderate exercise and the emotional support required to achieve the goal.

CPSIA information can be obtained
at www.ICGtesting.com
Printed in the USA
BVHW070856150321
602550BV00010B/1195